I0791449

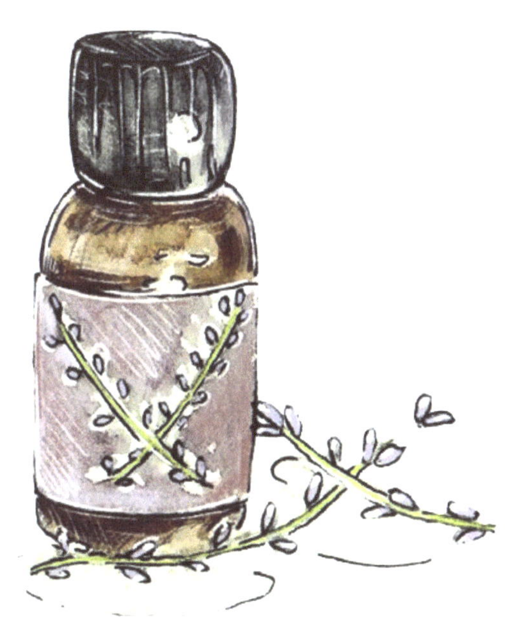

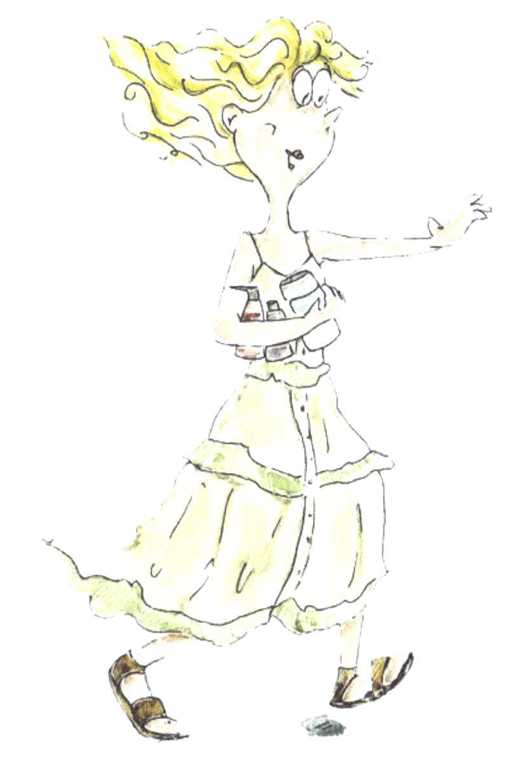

MUM'S SPECIAL OILS

By Cat Davies

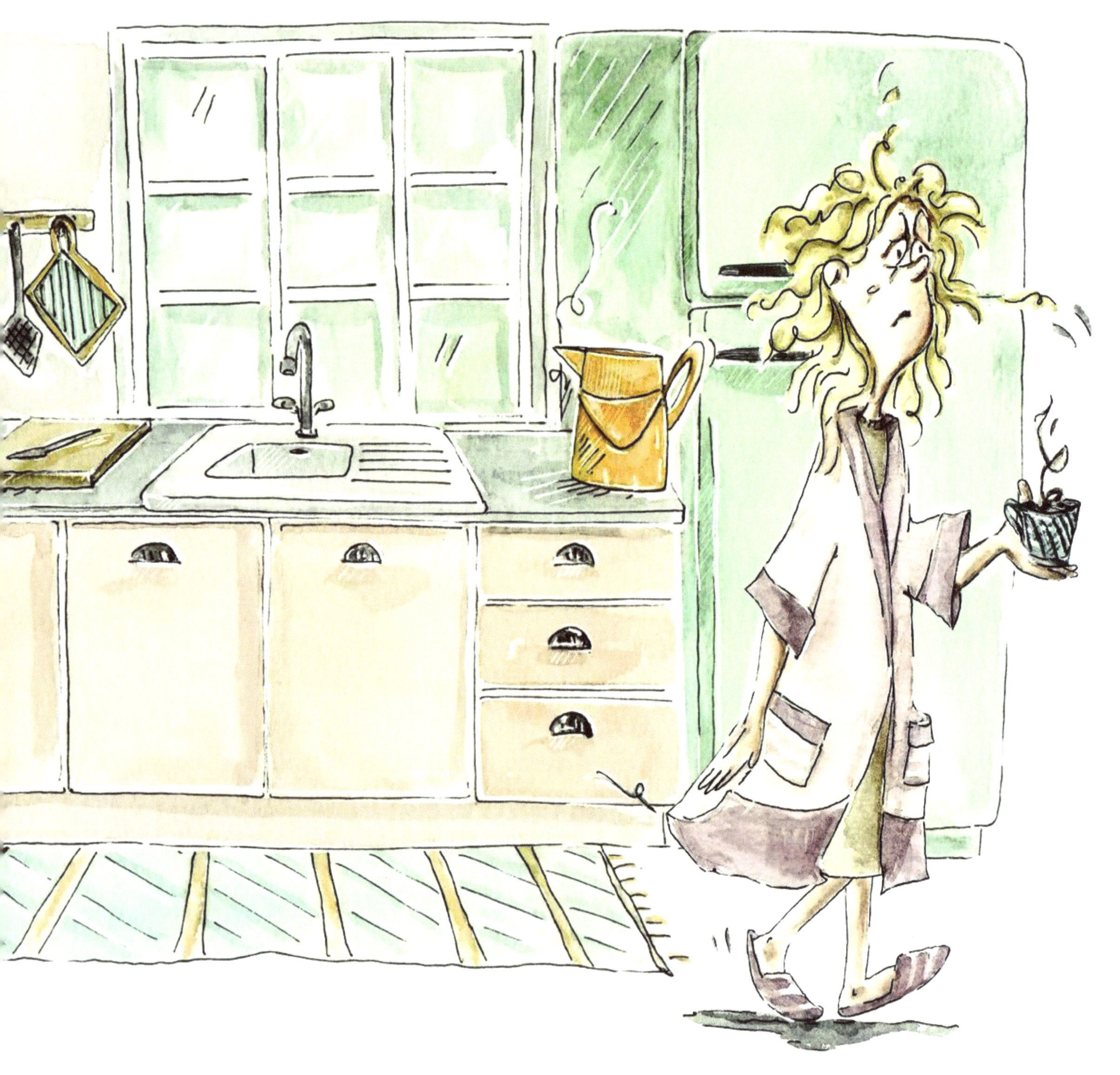

It was a typical day when things went amiss.
It started with my Mum, and it went like this.

Mum had not slept well; she'd tossed and turned all night.
When she crawled into the kitchen, she really looked a fright.

She was super grumpy too, stomping all about,
That's when she decided to try essential oils out.

That night she used Lavender oil to help her get some sleep.
The next morning she said, "I slept all night without a peep!"

"It's amazing, it's wonderful! I want to try some more."
And the very next morning the Postman was at our door.

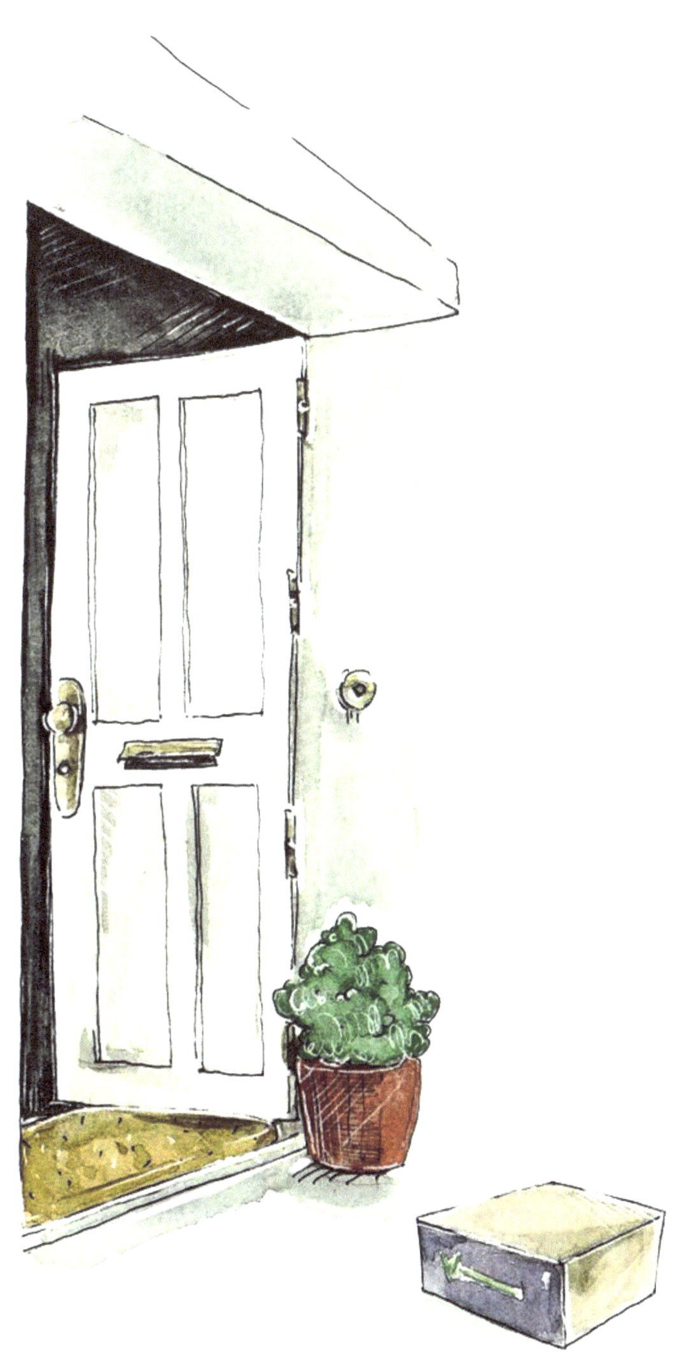

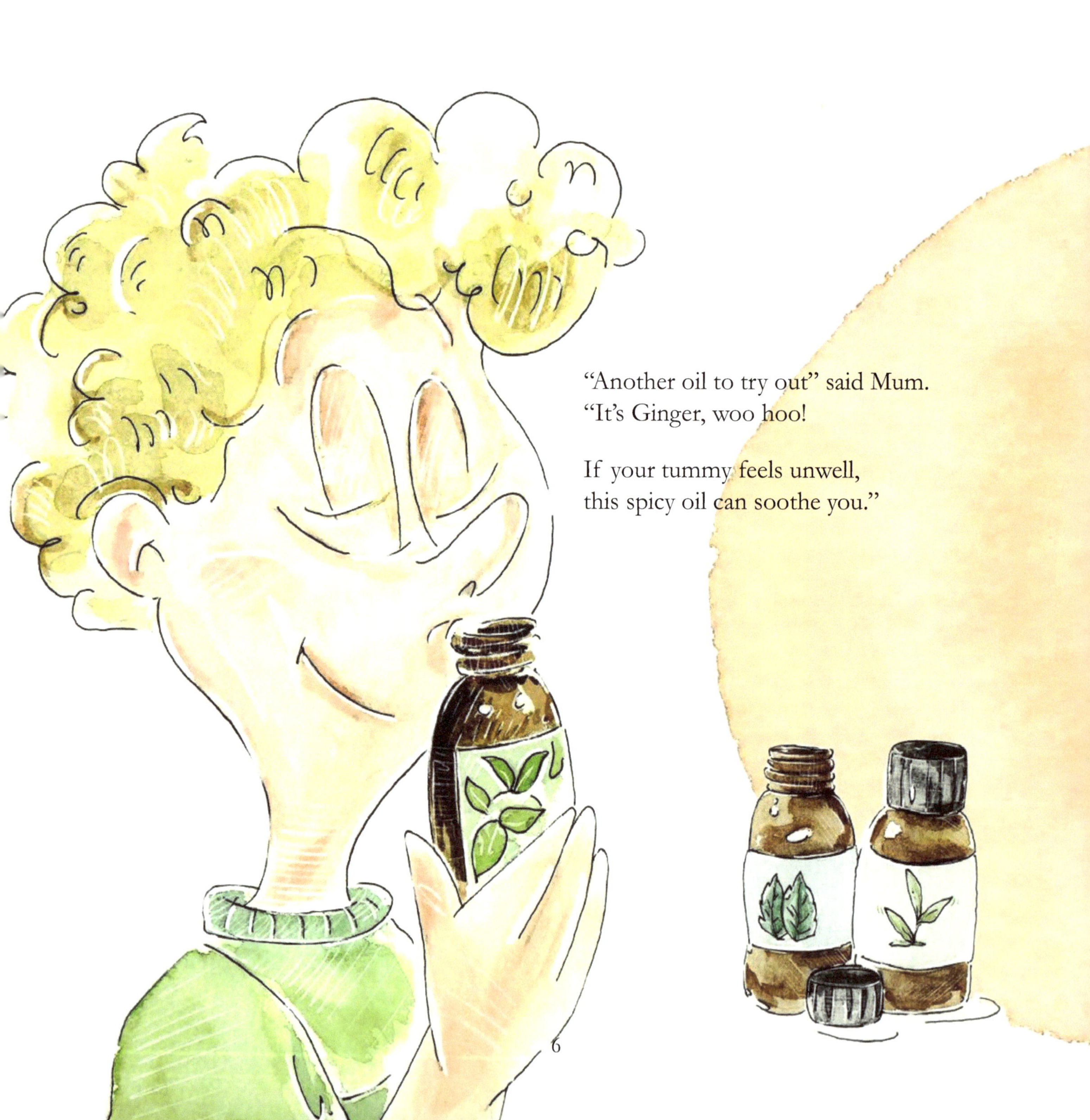

"Another oil to try out" said Mum.
"It's Ginger, woo hoo!

If your tummy feels unwell,
this spicy oil can soothe you."

6

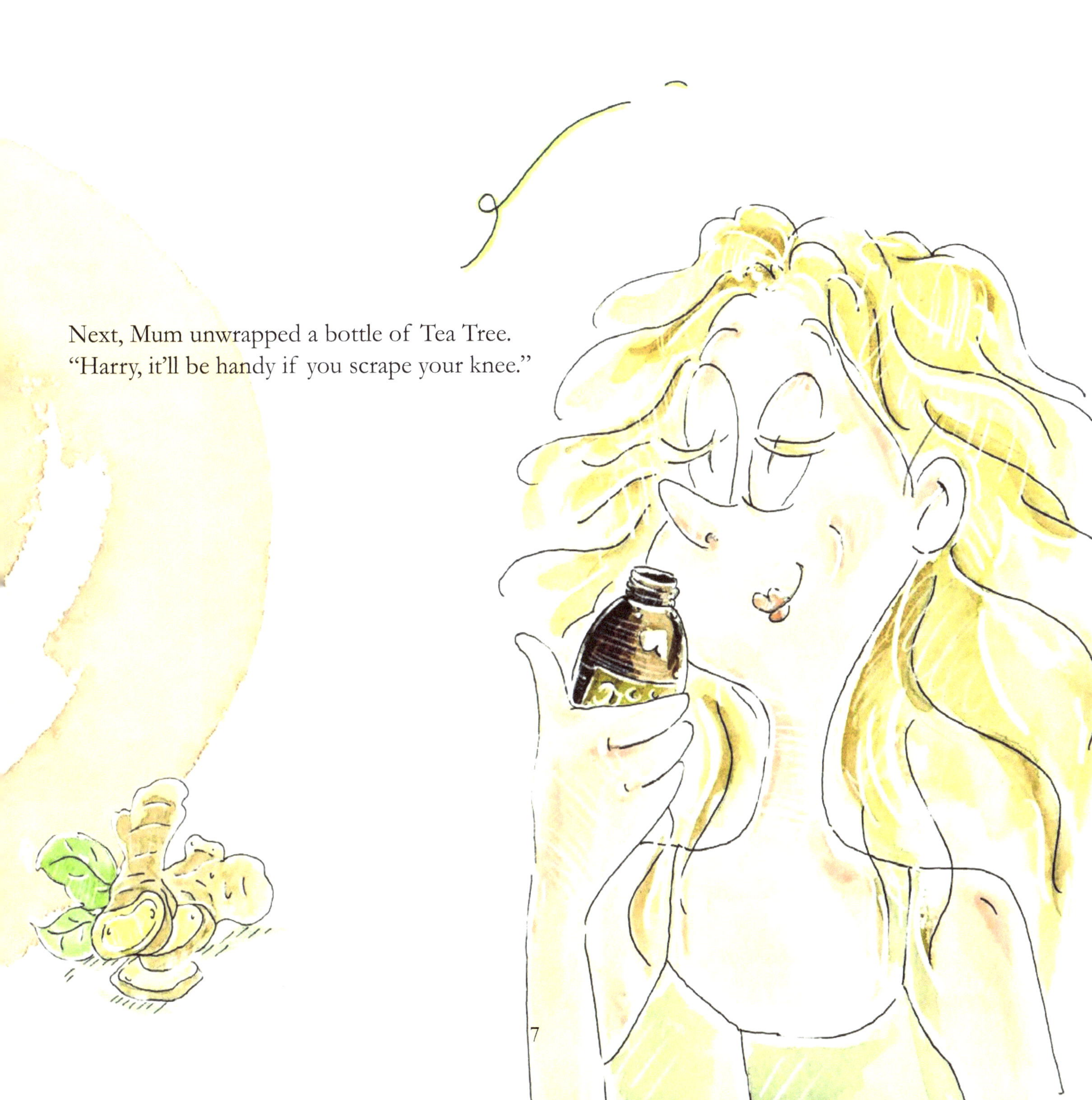

Next, Mum unwrapped a bottle of Tea Tree.
"Harry, it'll be handy if you scrape your knee."

I watched as Mum placed diffusers in every room.
Dad said our home now smelled of nothing but perfume.

Mum said, "Oh, I love my oils, and want to try some more"...

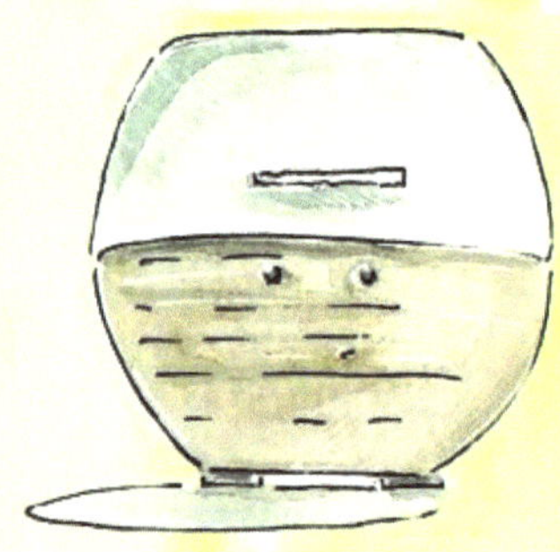

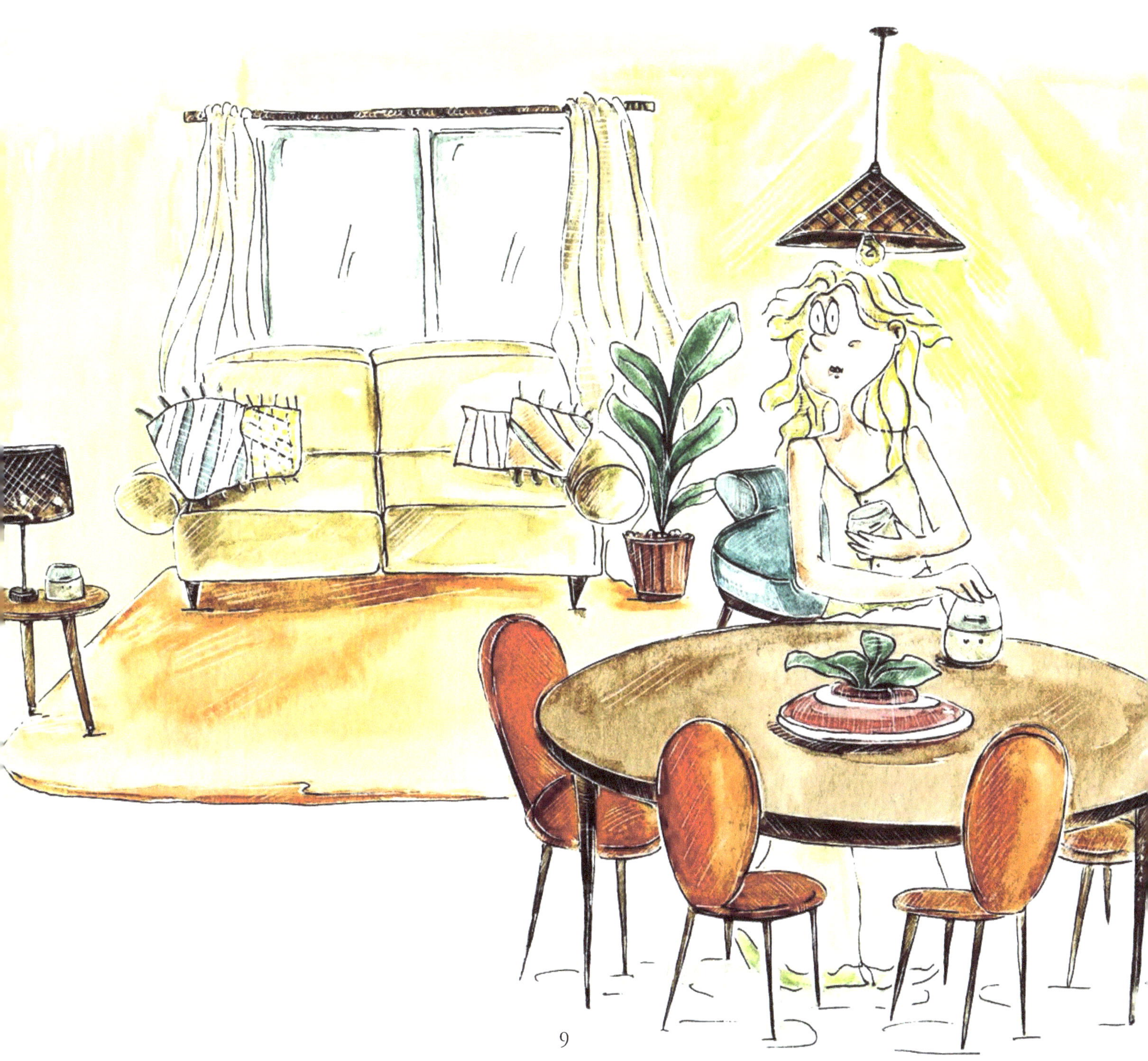

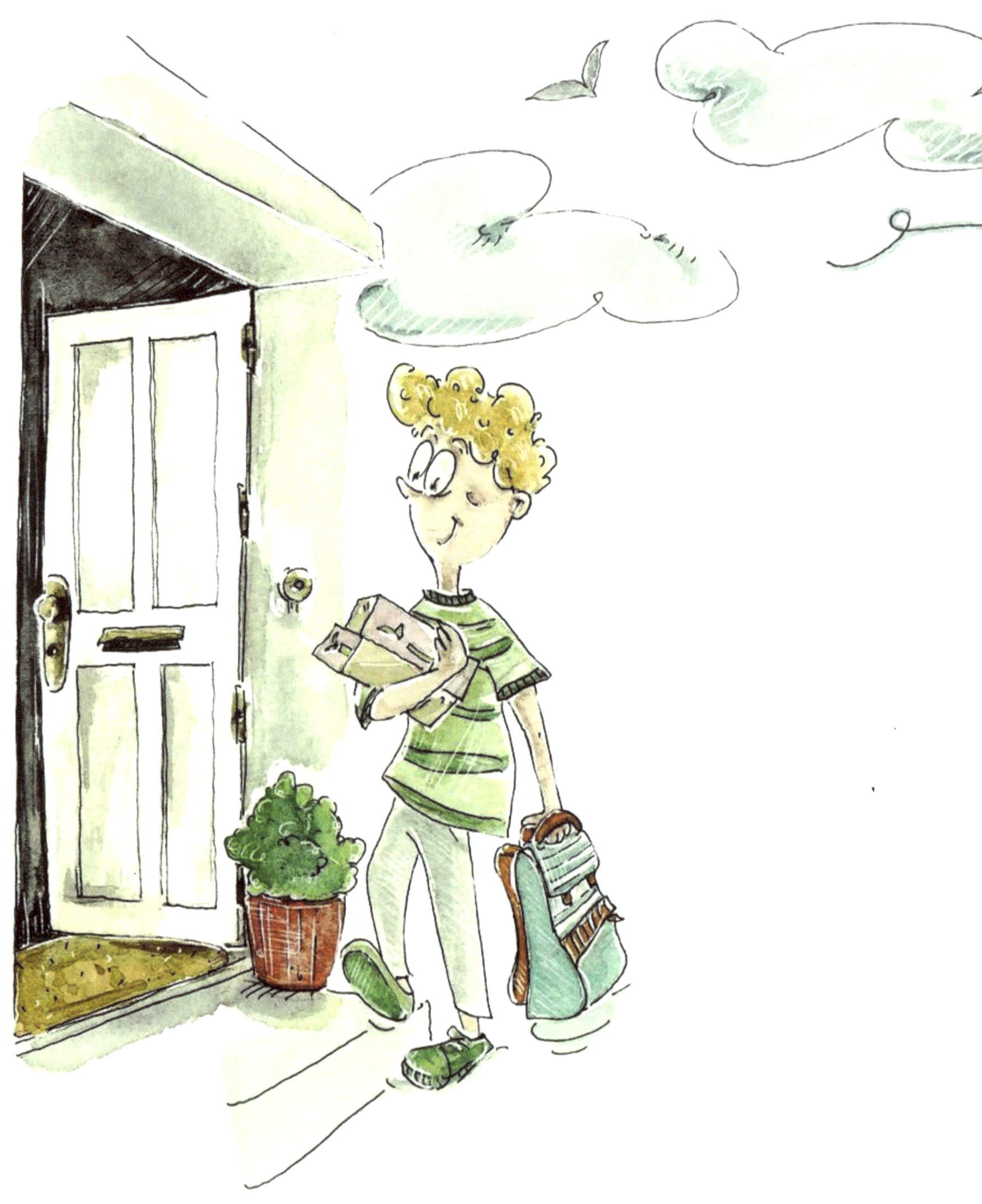

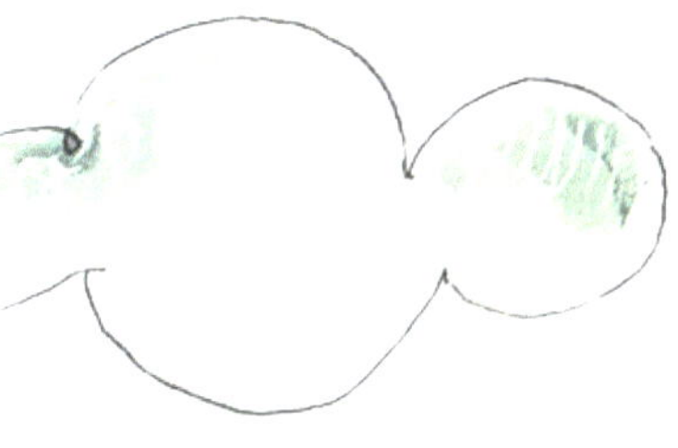

And soon there was another package left at the door!

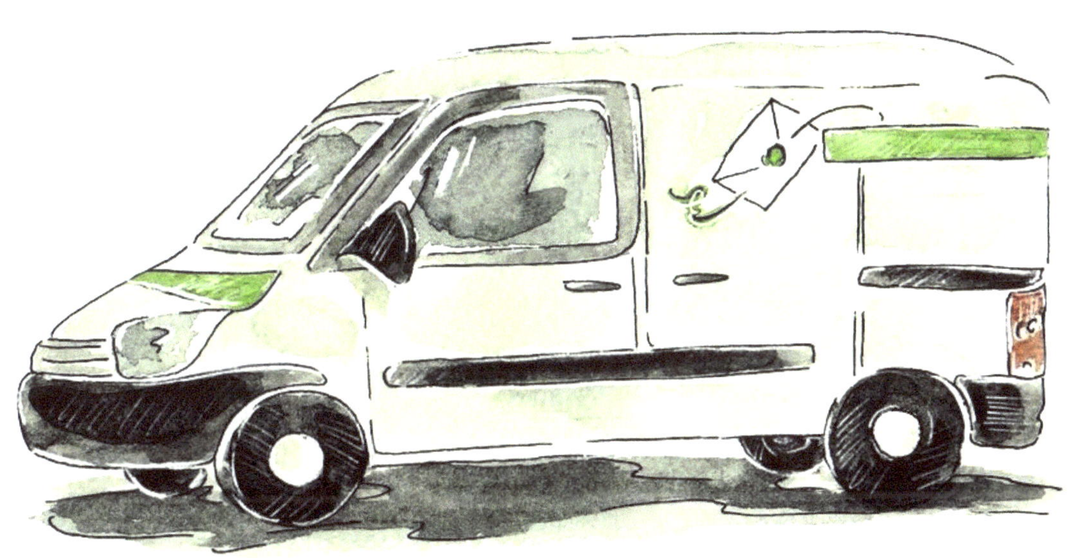

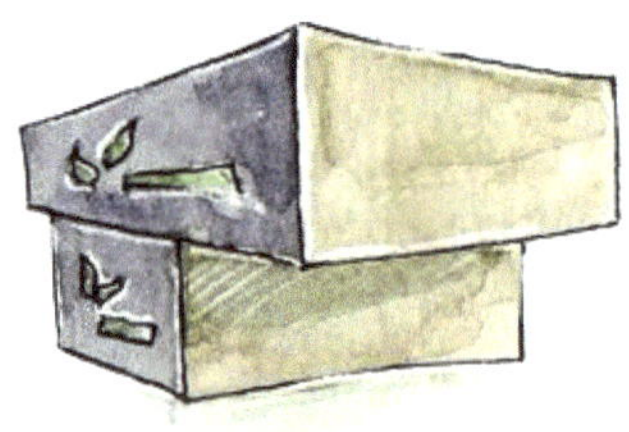

"What is it this time?" said Dad, his eyes rolling up to the sky
"It's rose oil for making soap" exclaimed Mum with a happy cry!

Dad walked away and scoffed at all of Mum's 'oohs' and 'aahs,'
But I thought it smelled nice, like the flowers at Grandma's.

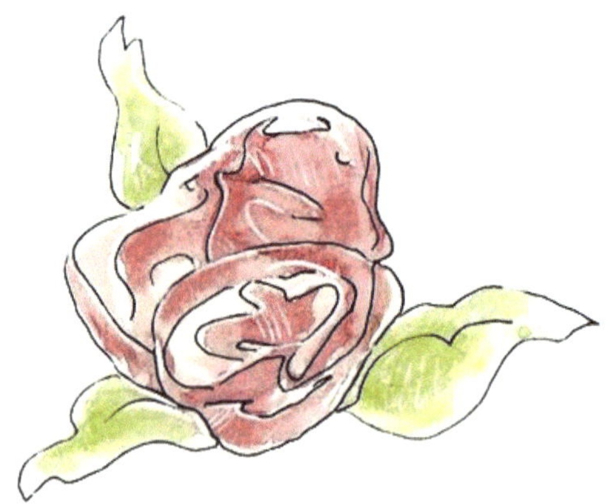

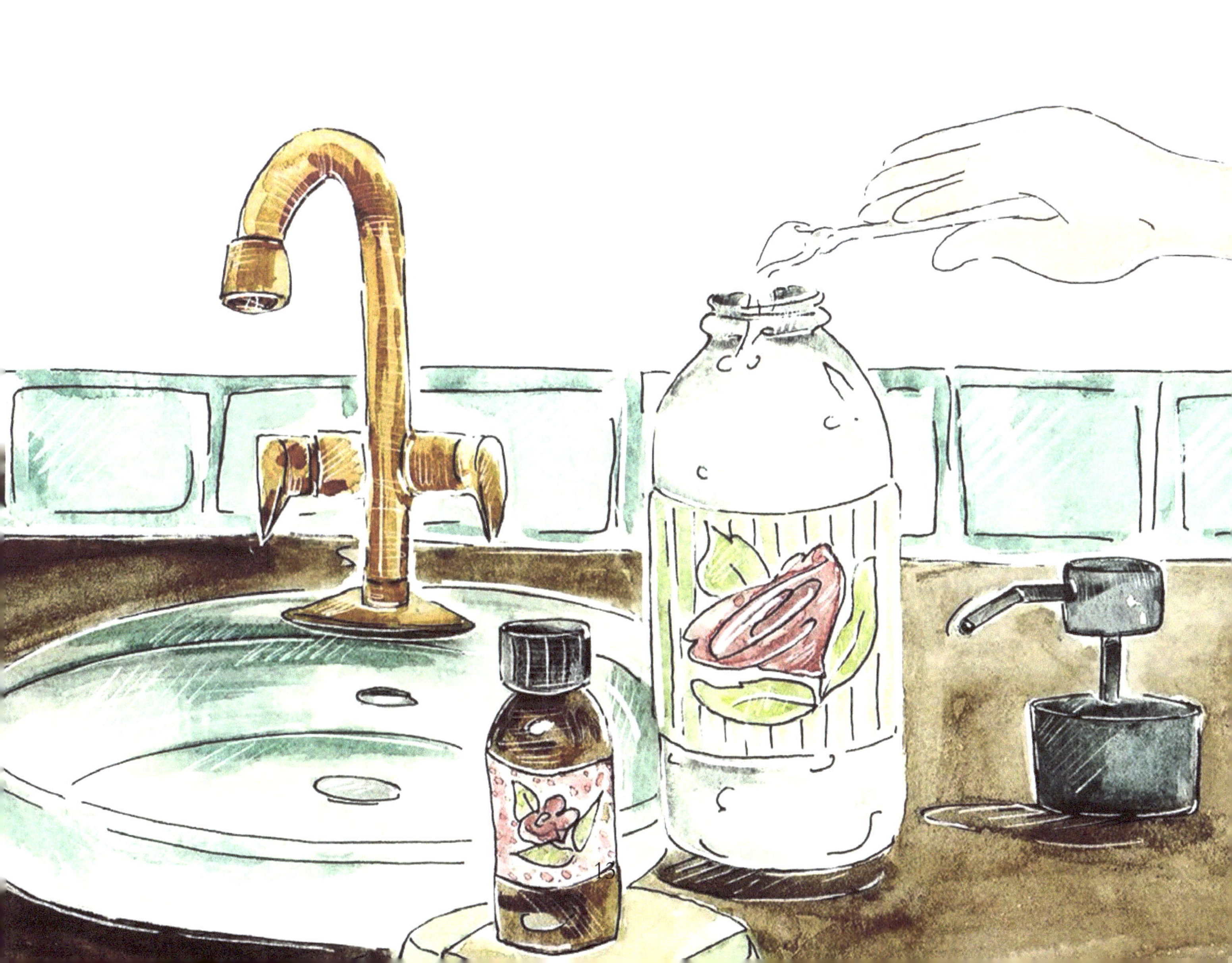

13

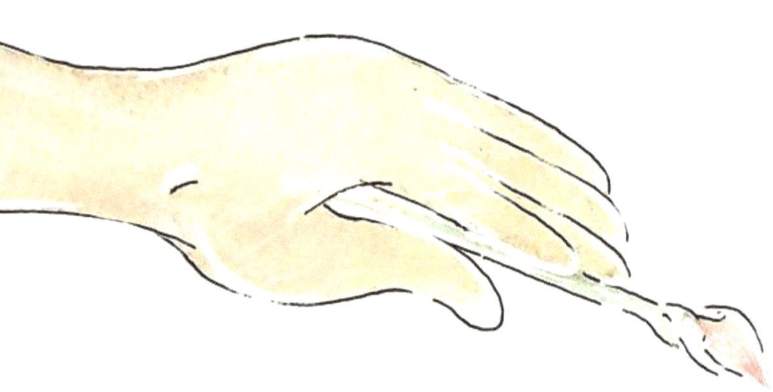

Later I washed my hands with Mum's homemade rose soap.

It was pretty good I thought, and that thought gave me hope...

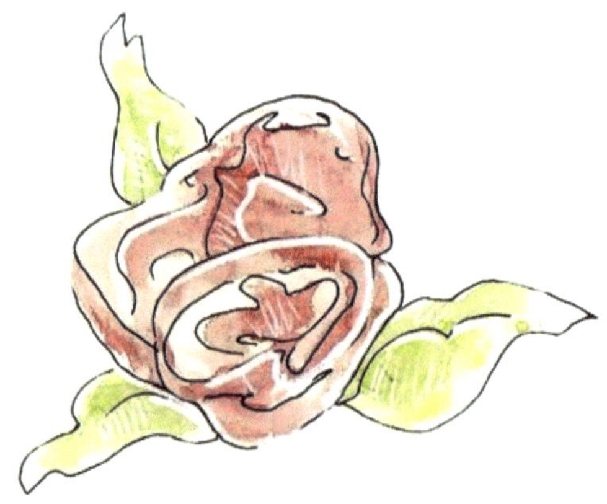

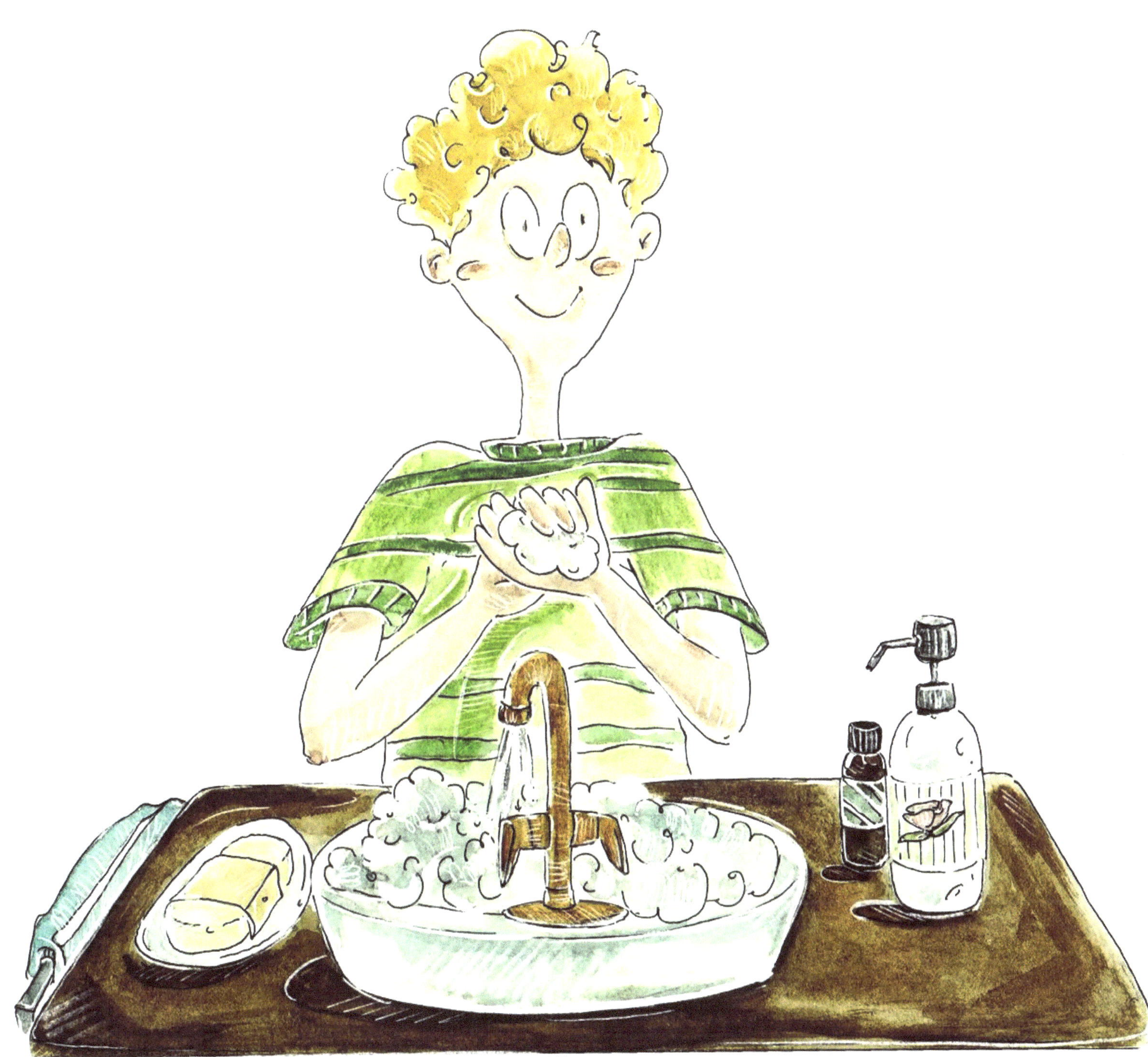

Maybe Mum's oil obsession wasn't so bad after all.
But then I heard a knock and Mum running down the hall.

The postman here again? Oh no, it couldn't be!
"I'm coming" cried Mum. "That parcel is for me!"

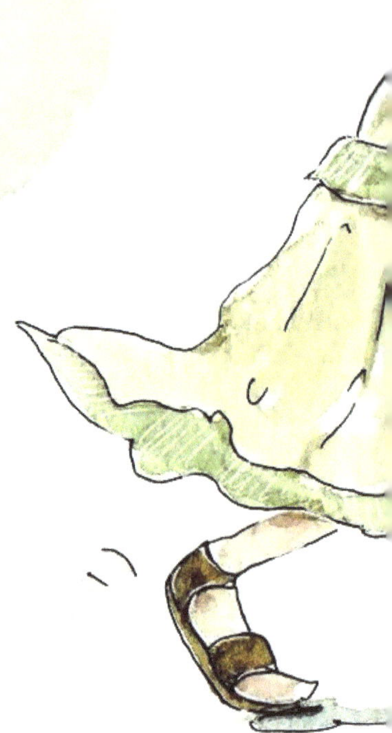

16

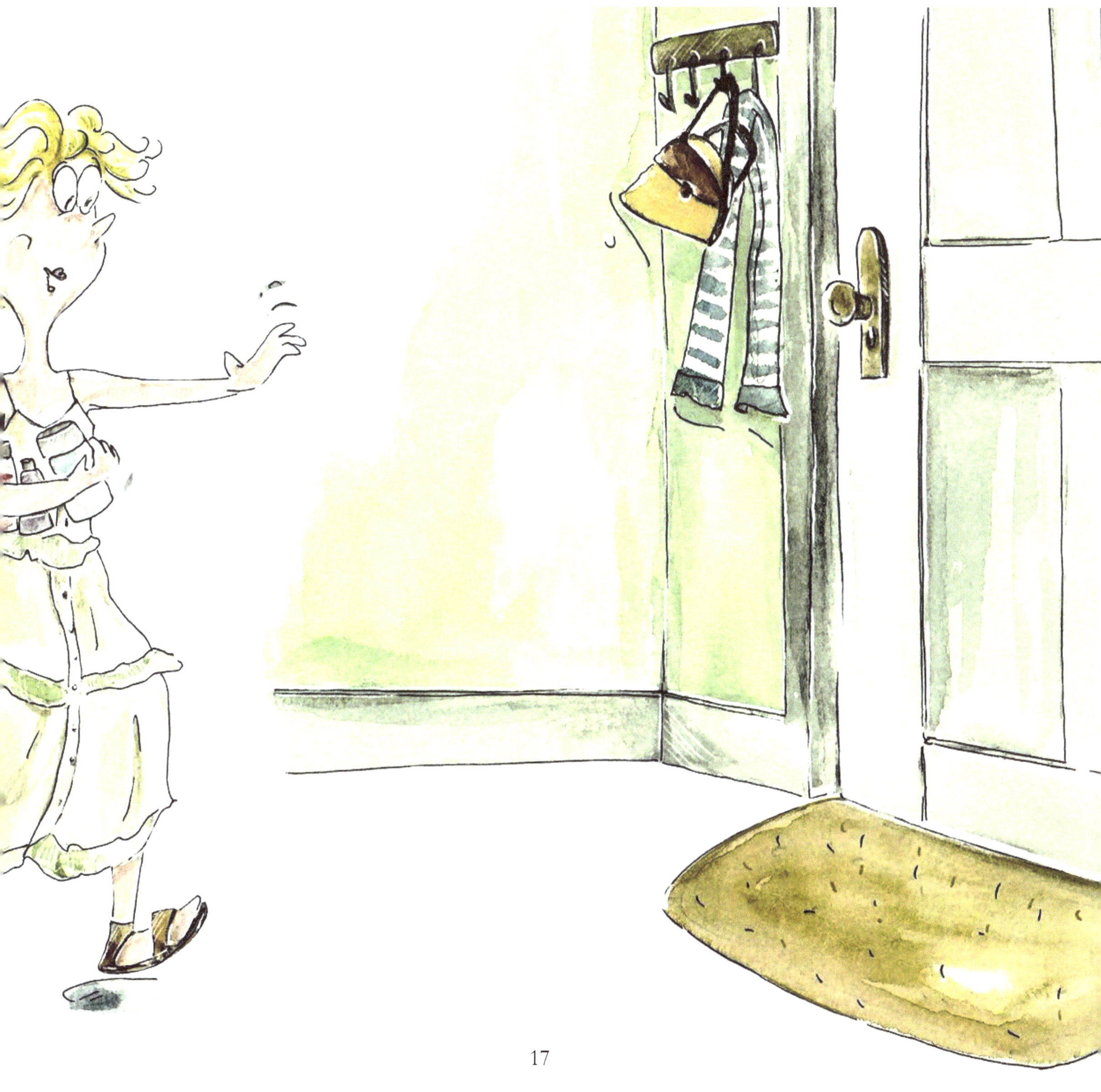

Later a racket in the kitchen made Dad ask, "What's happening now?"
"Ohh I think she's making something yummy - Mum, can you show me how?"

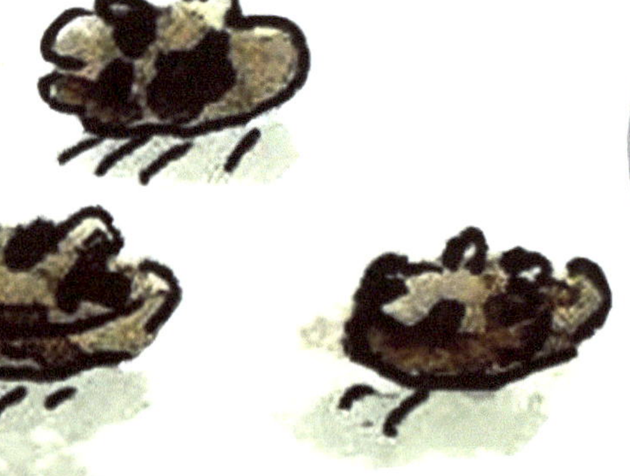

"Thank you, Harry. I will mix while you add a special drop.
These gooey peppermint brownies will make your taste buds pop!"

The brownies sure did taste good; I managed to devour four!

Mum said, "The rest are for my oil party, so don't eat any more!"

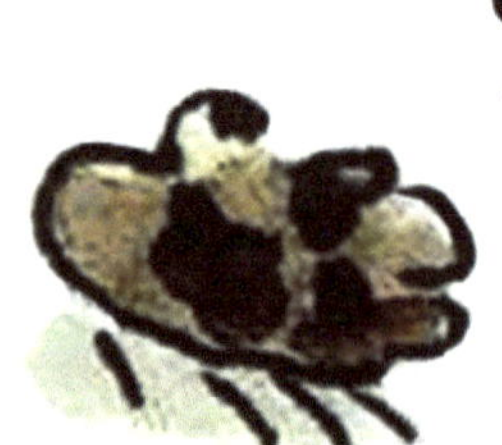

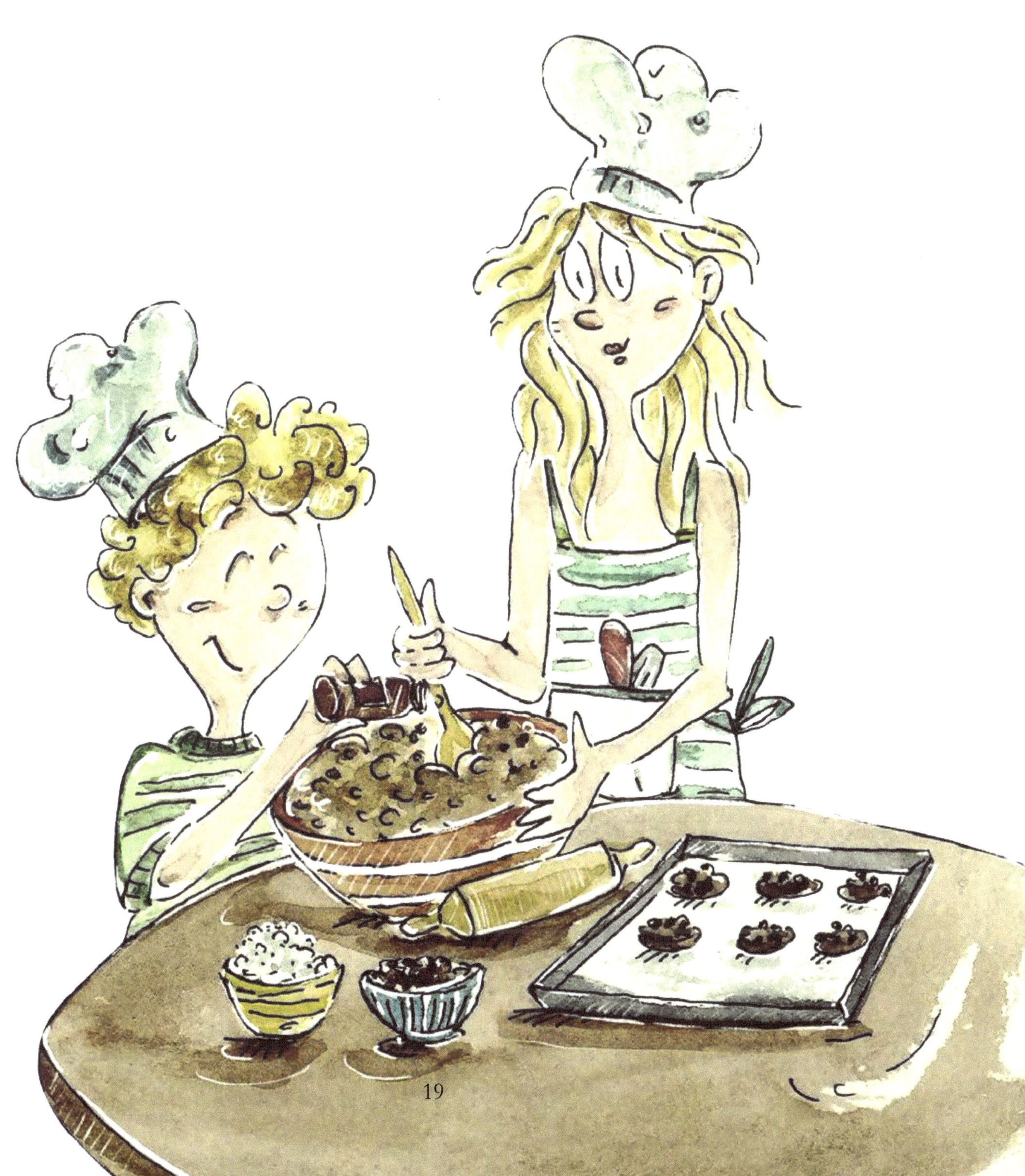

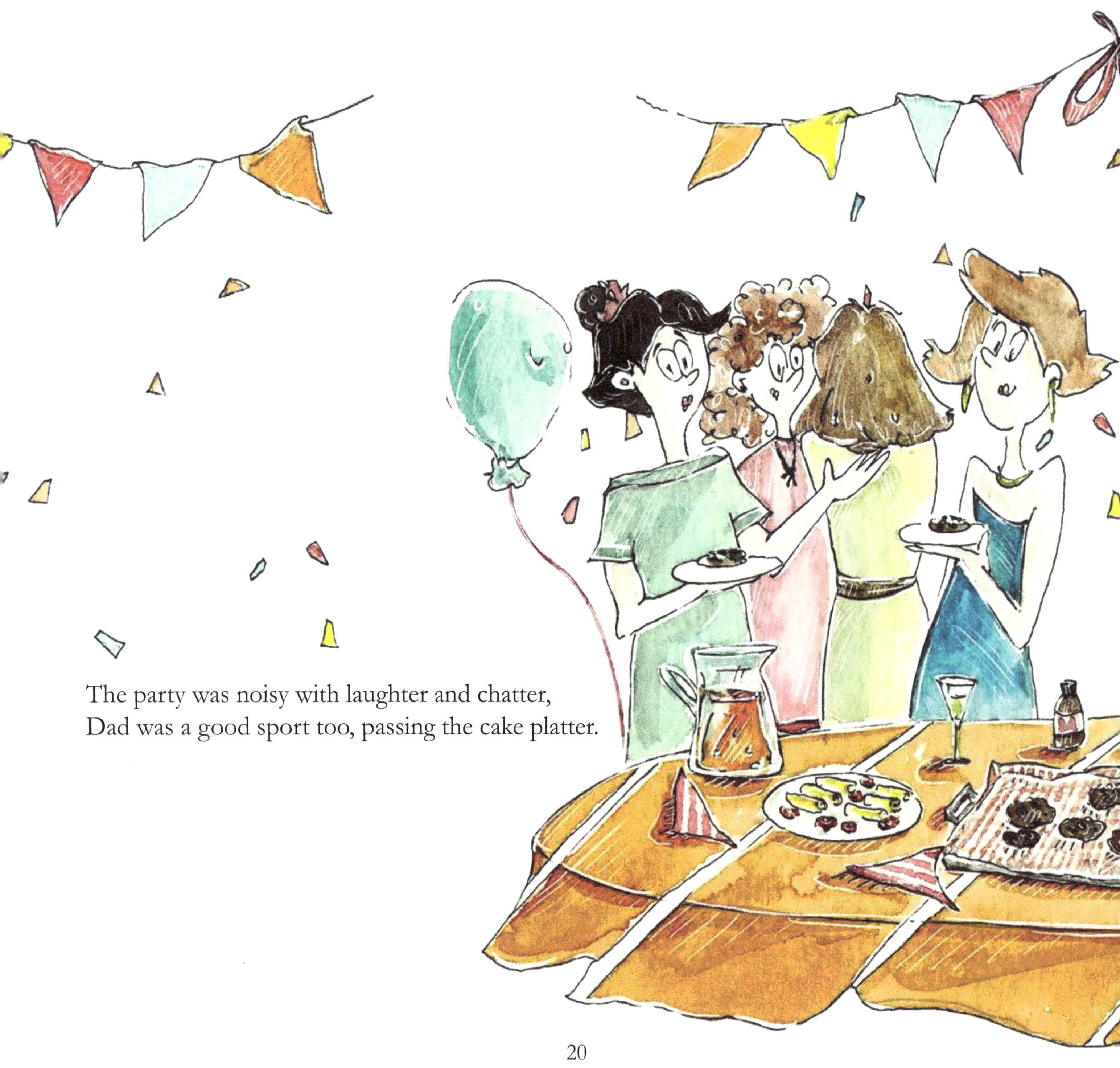

The party was noisy with laughter and chatter,
Dad was a good sport too, passing the cake platter.

20

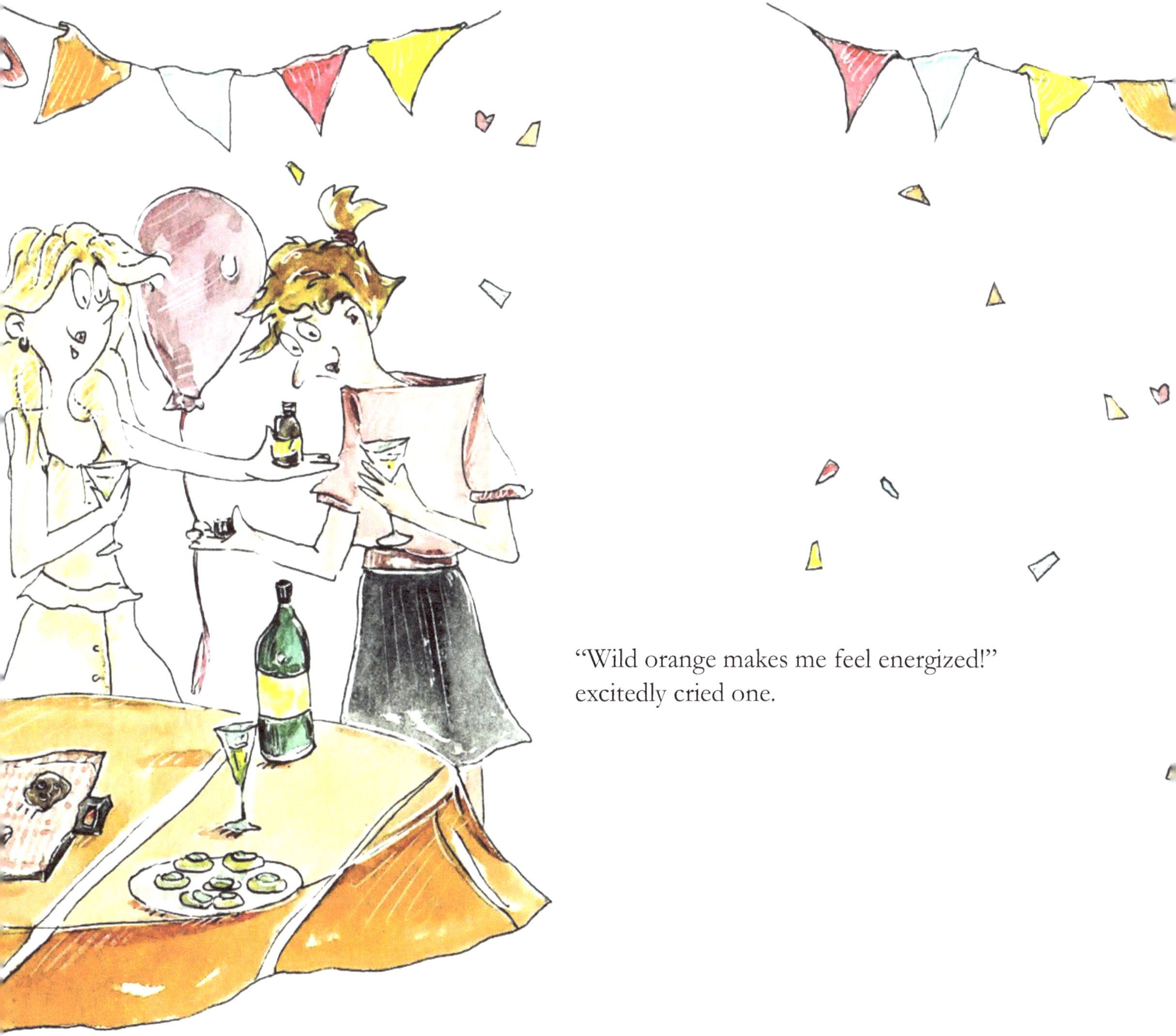

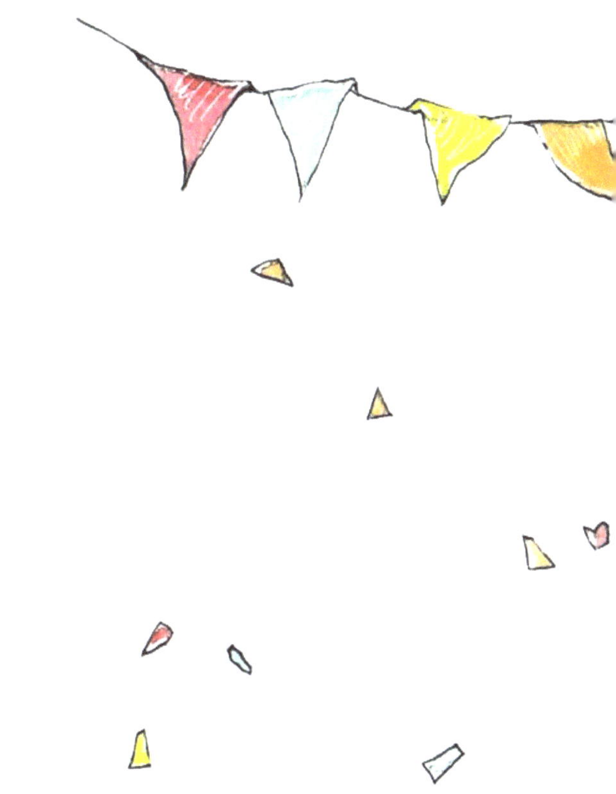

"Wild orange makes me feel energized!" excitedly cried one.

"You must try the magnolia in a bath bomb," suggested Mum.

"If you've had a particularly horrid day,
Pop one in your bath to help worries drift away"

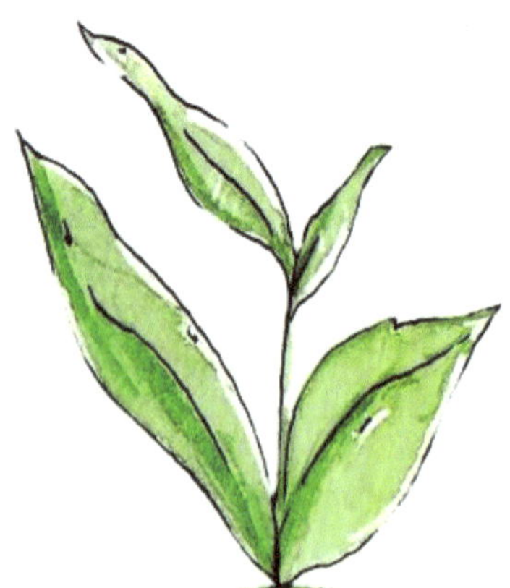

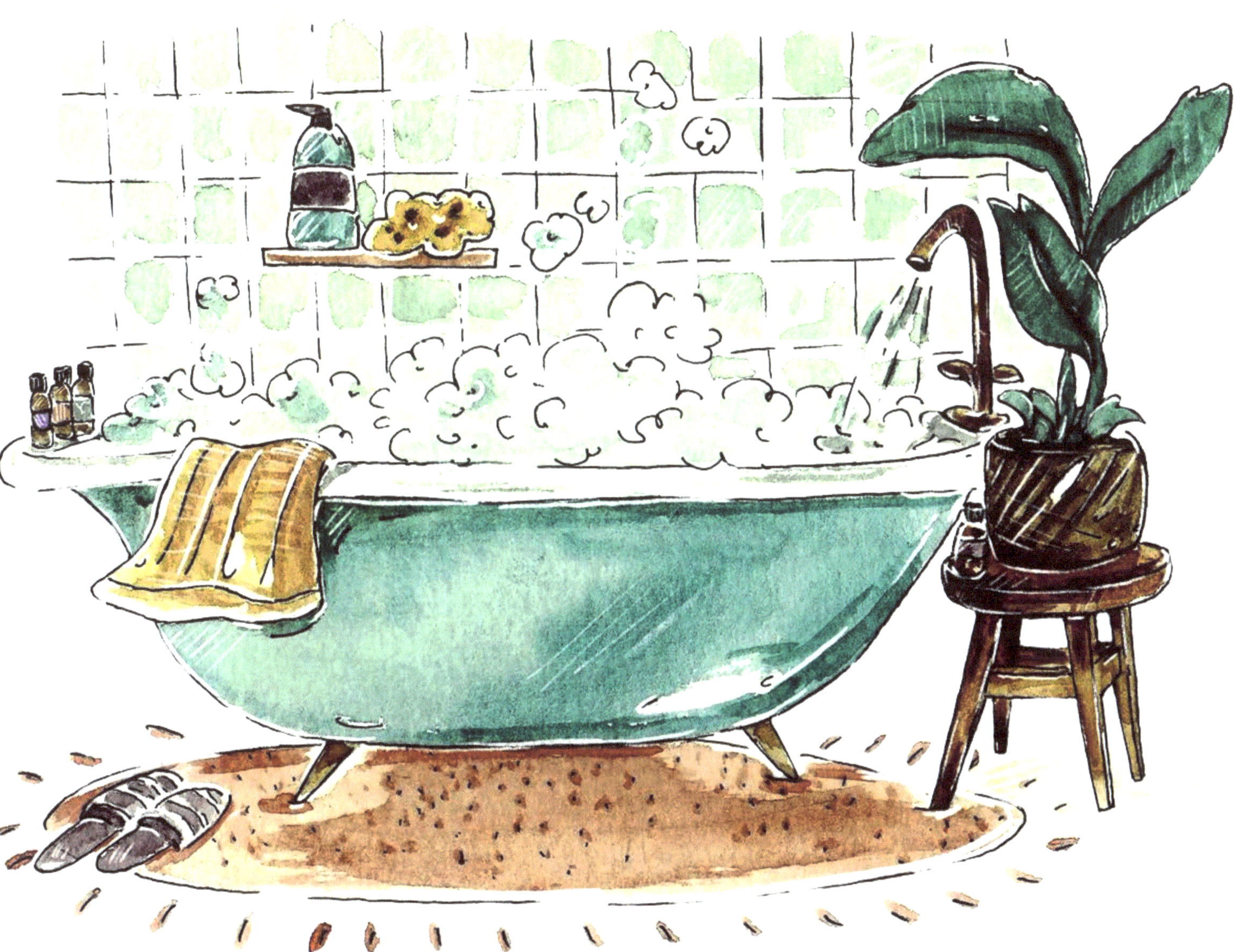

The next morning I was nervous about my English test.
Mum said, "Try some Frankincense, it really is the best.

You may think that I'm crazy, but try it, anyway?"
"Sure, Mum," I replied, itching to get on with my day.

Mum got busy again, mixing up her 'calm balm'.
"Come here" she said "I'll put a little on your arm."

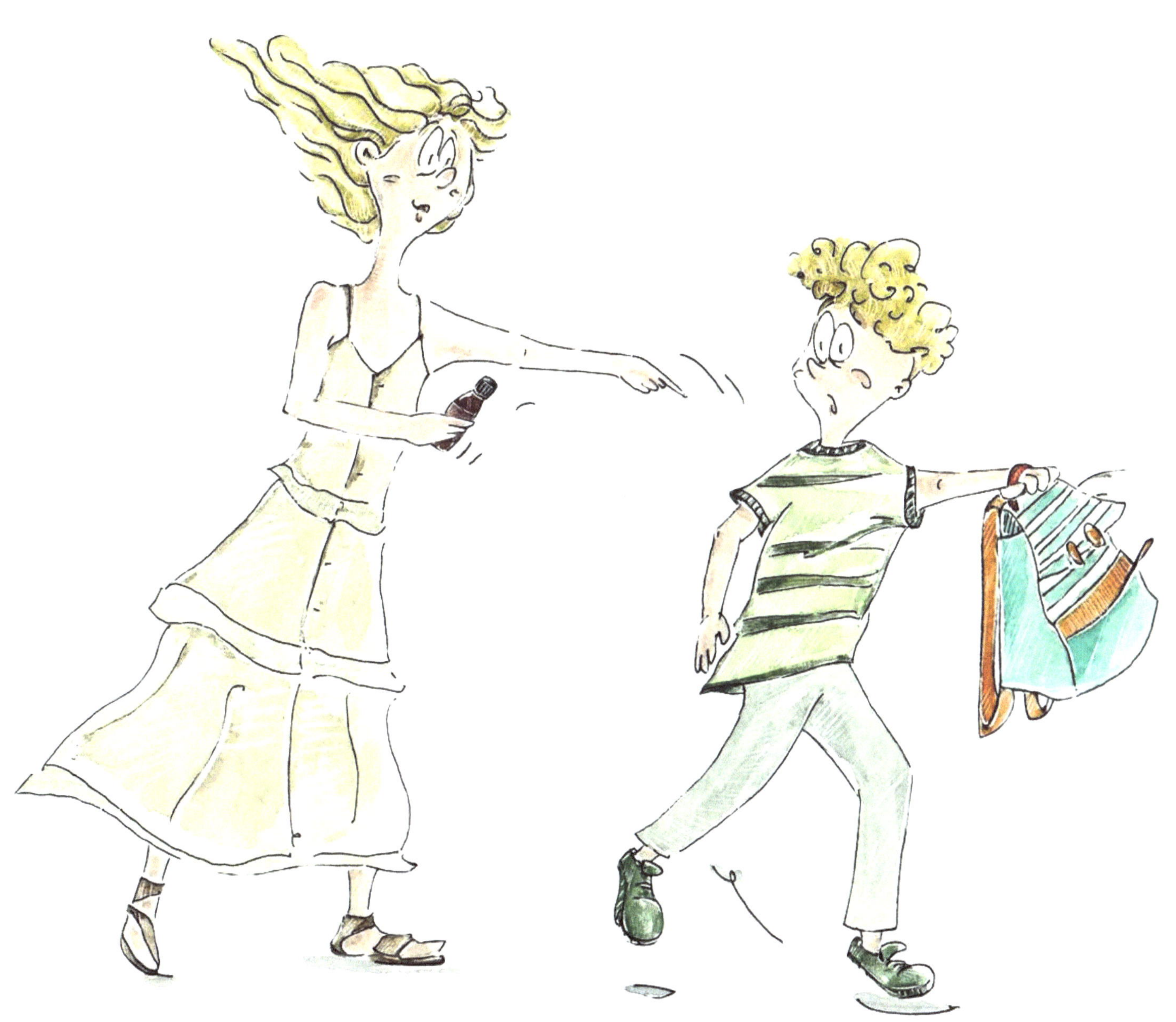

I shook my head and thought, My mates will think I'm such a fool,
But I found myself enjoying the woody oil at school!

I imagined I was in a forest, swinging gently from a tree.
I felt so calm and cosy but most of all completely carefree.

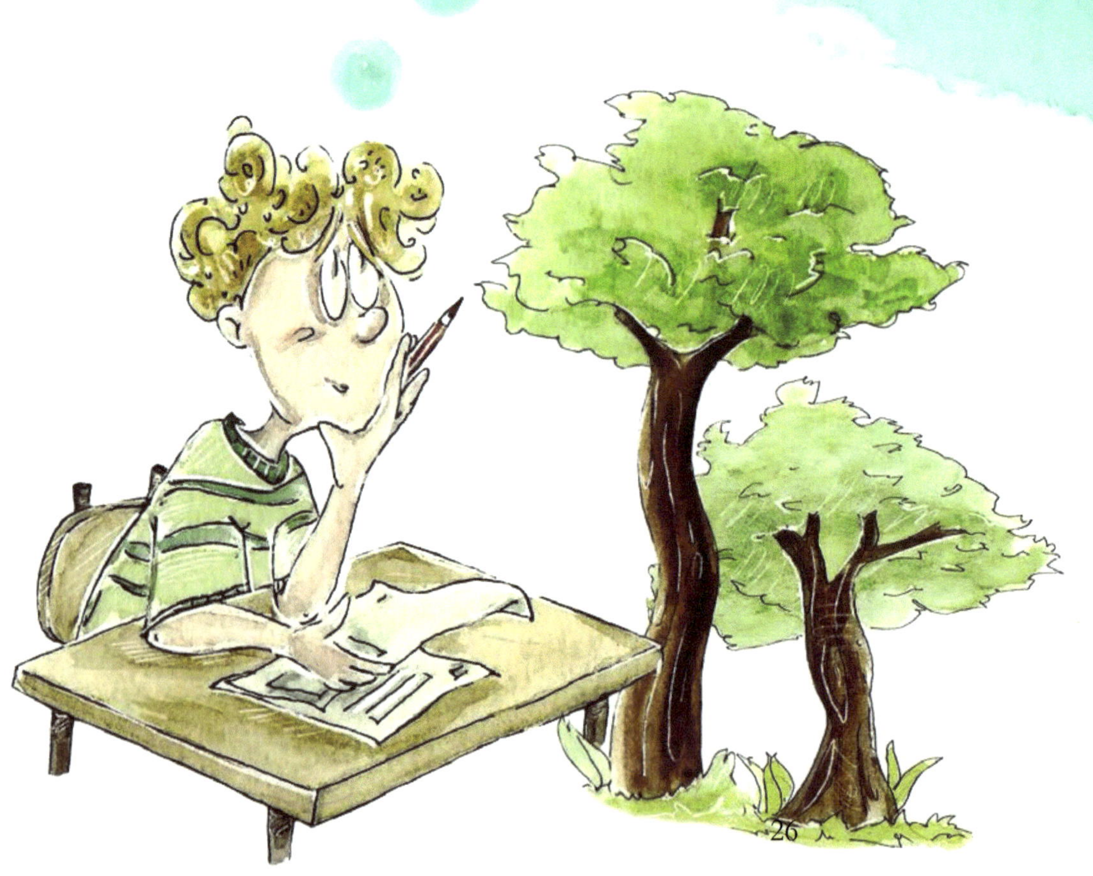

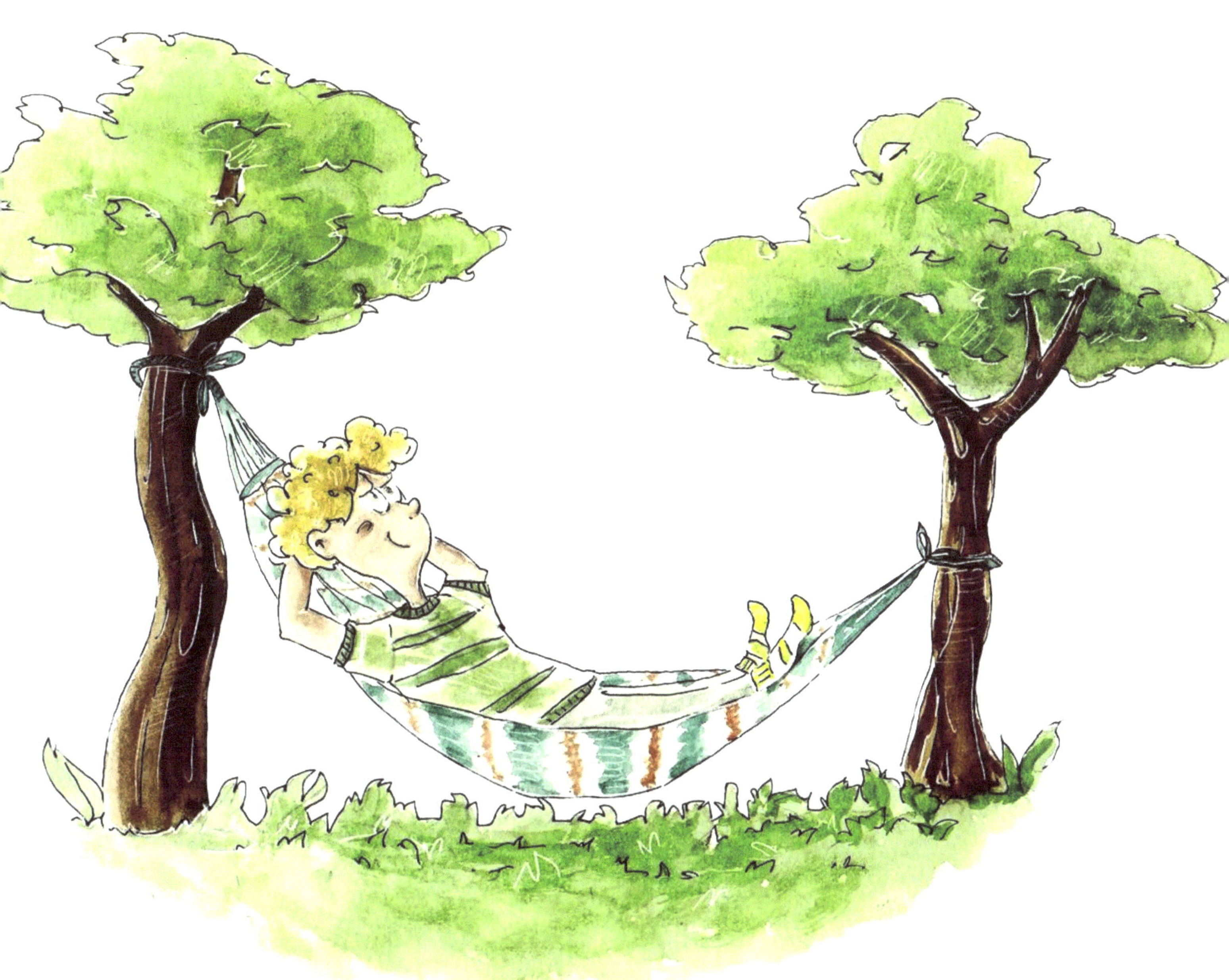

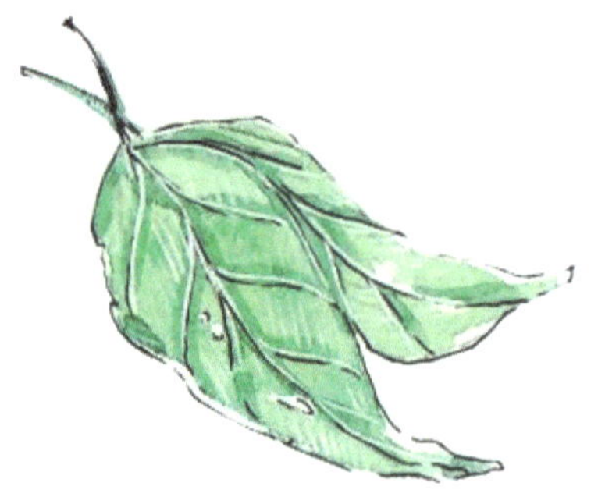

Dad collapsed into the kitchen from his evening run.

I said, "Dad, I don't know why you think running so far is fun!"

"It's great" said Dad "but after my legs lose all their zing."

"Wait right there," called Mum. "I think I may have just the thing!"

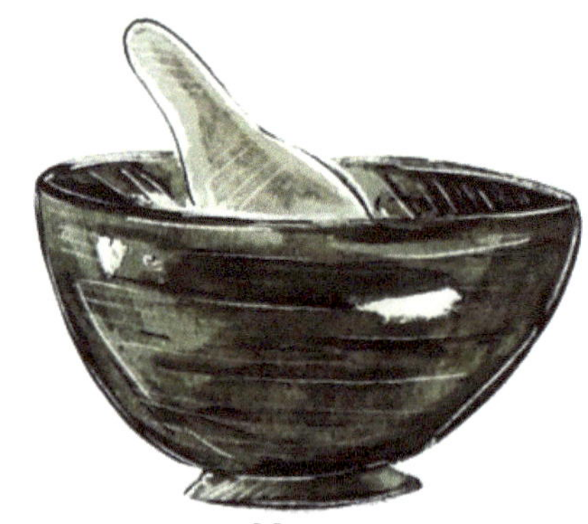

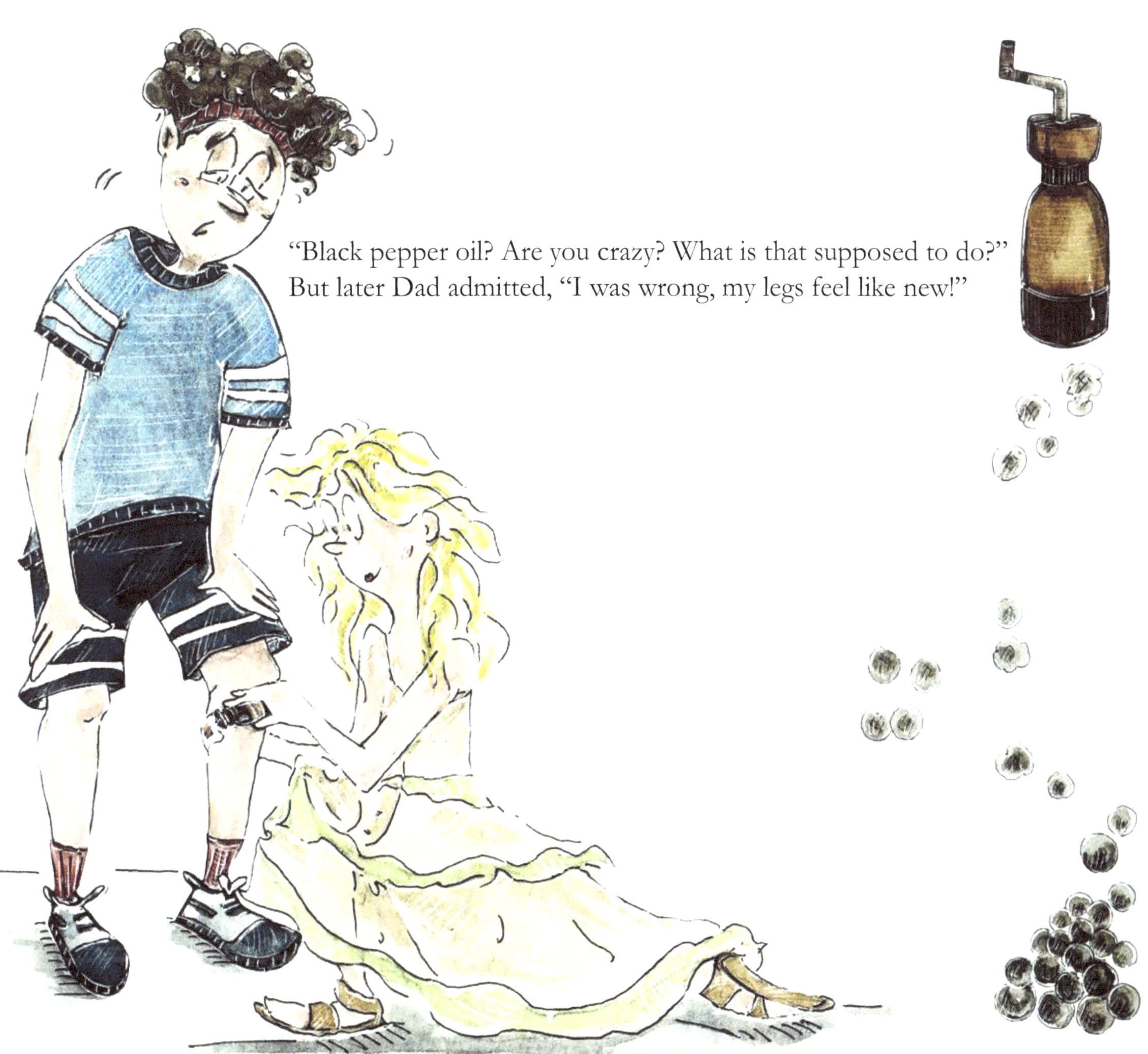

"Black pepper oil? Are you crazy? What is that supposed to do?"
But later Dad admitted, "I was wrong, my legs feel like new!"

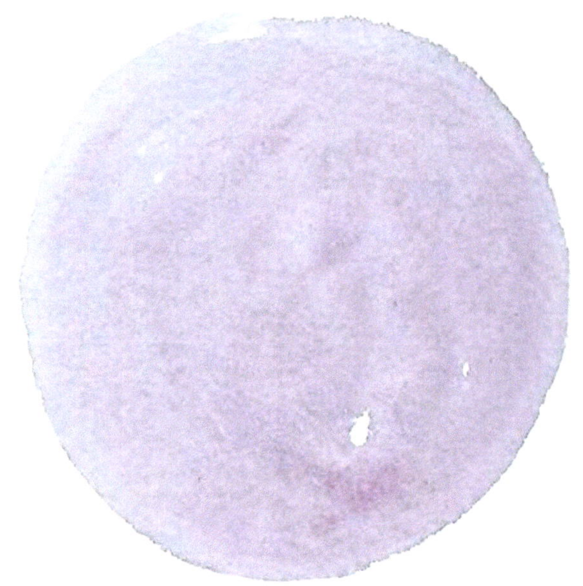

That night we all had foot baths. "Grab your oils!" suggested Dad.
We all agreed, it was the best foot bath we'd ever had.

Mum chose sweet Jasmine and Dad stinky Wintergreen,
I picked tangy Lime mixed with juicy Tangerine.

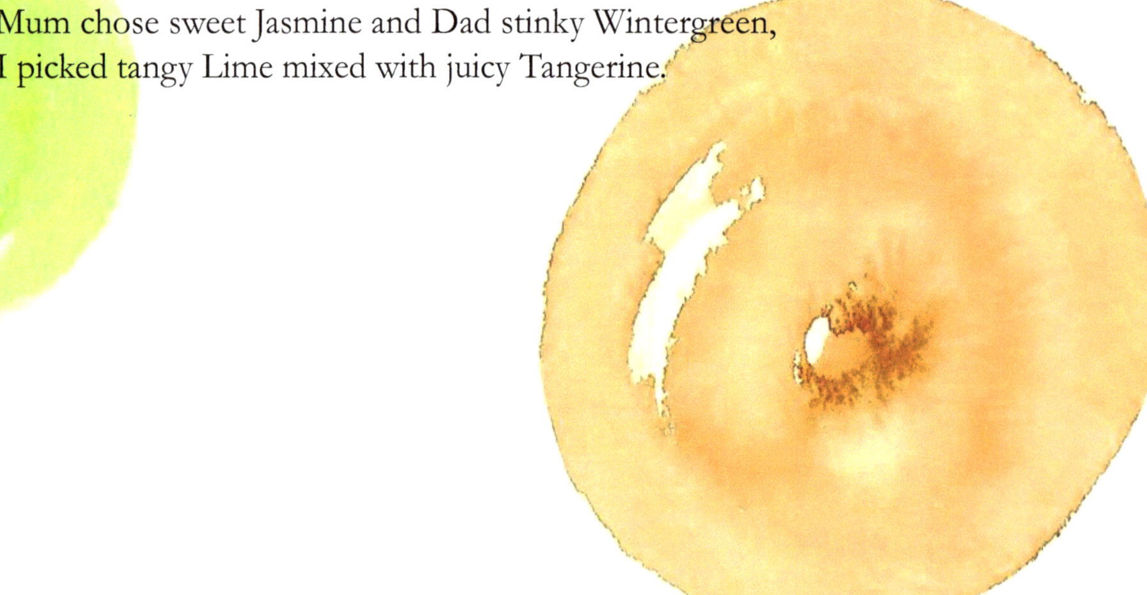

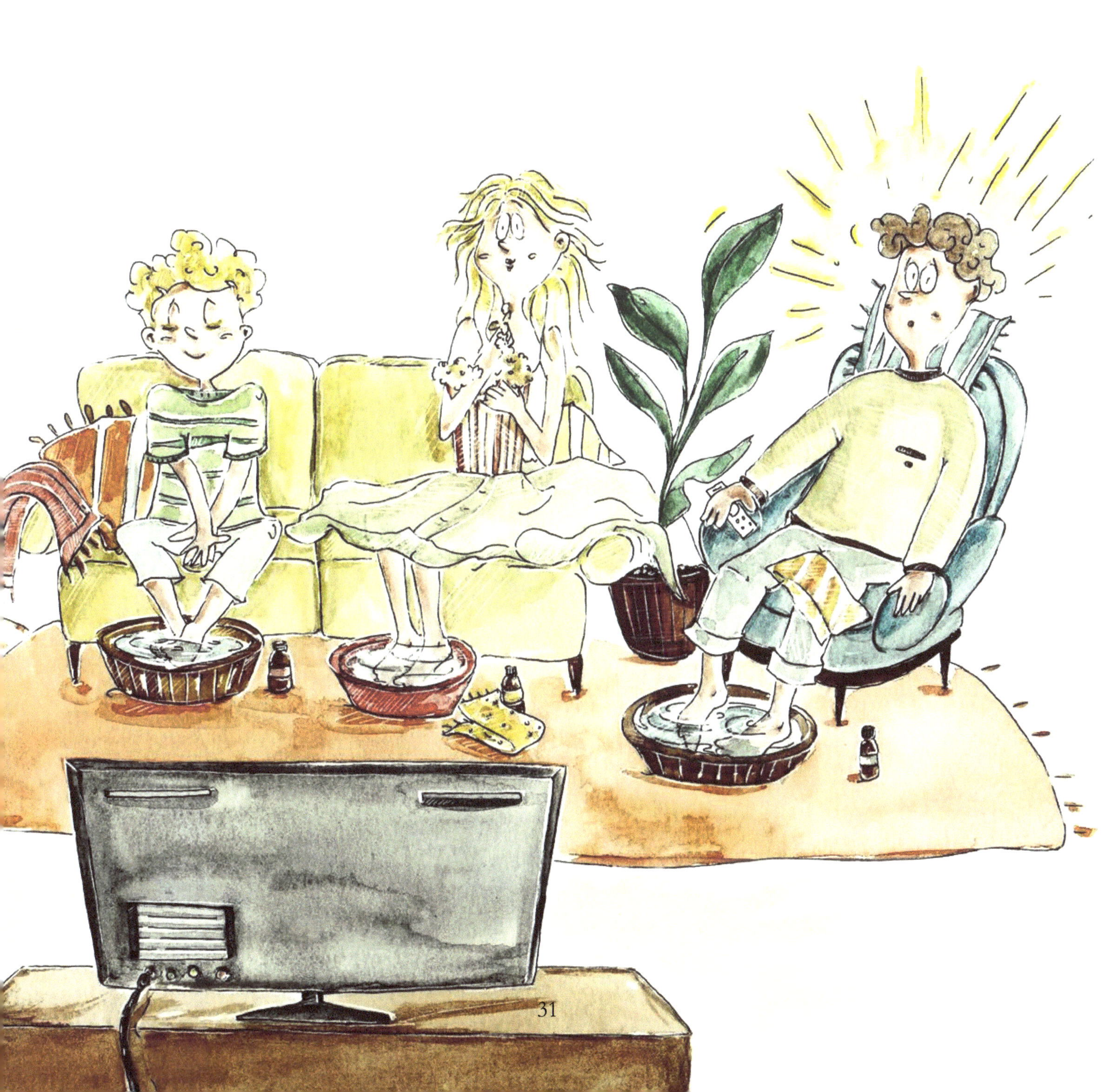

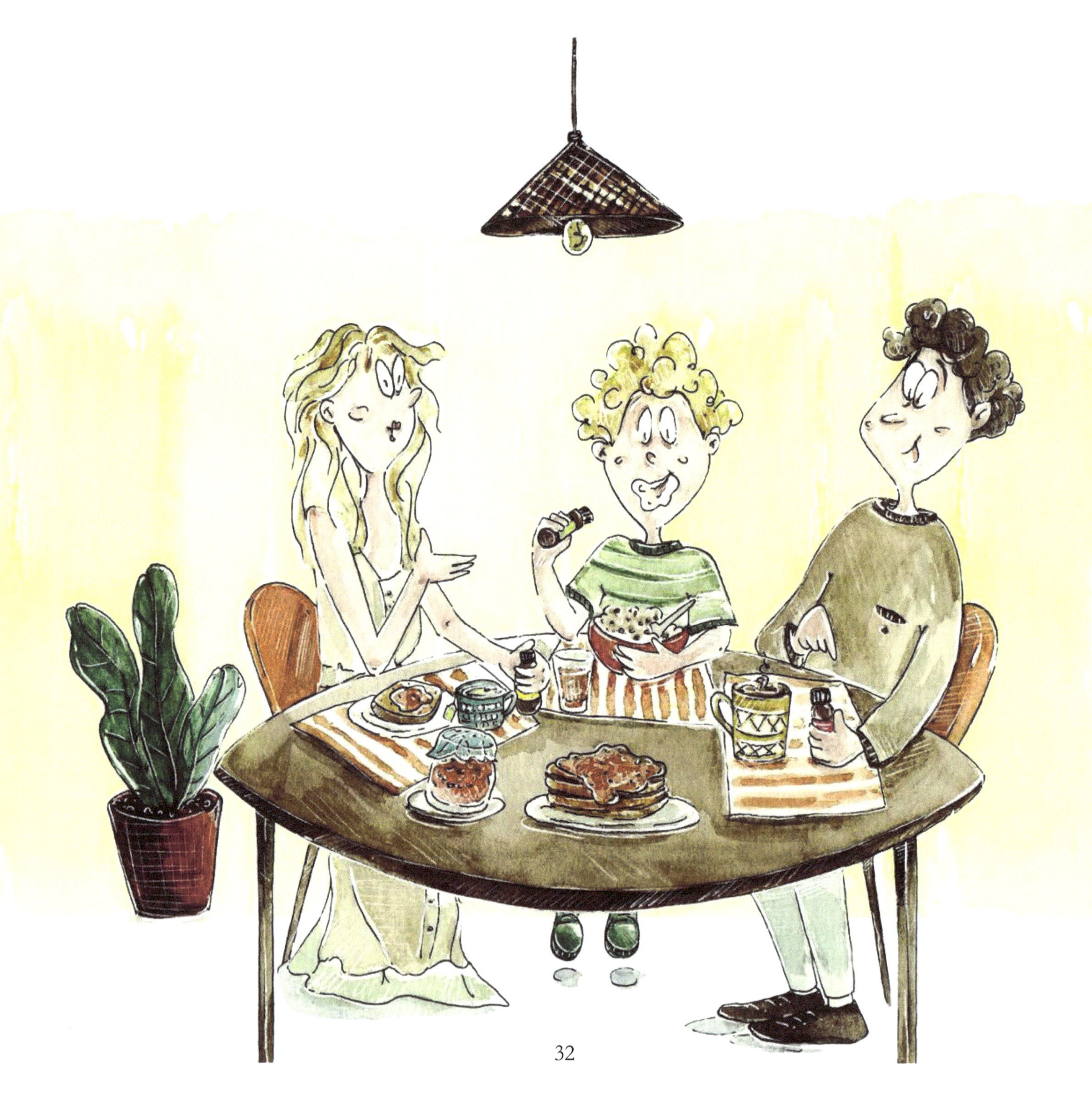

Next day at breakfast we ate wild orange marmalade on toast.

While Mum asked us which essential oil we liked the most.
I said, "I think Frankincense is by far the best"

"And Black Pepper is my favourite" Dad confessed

Mum began beaming from head to toe
And said she wished she had tried them years ago.

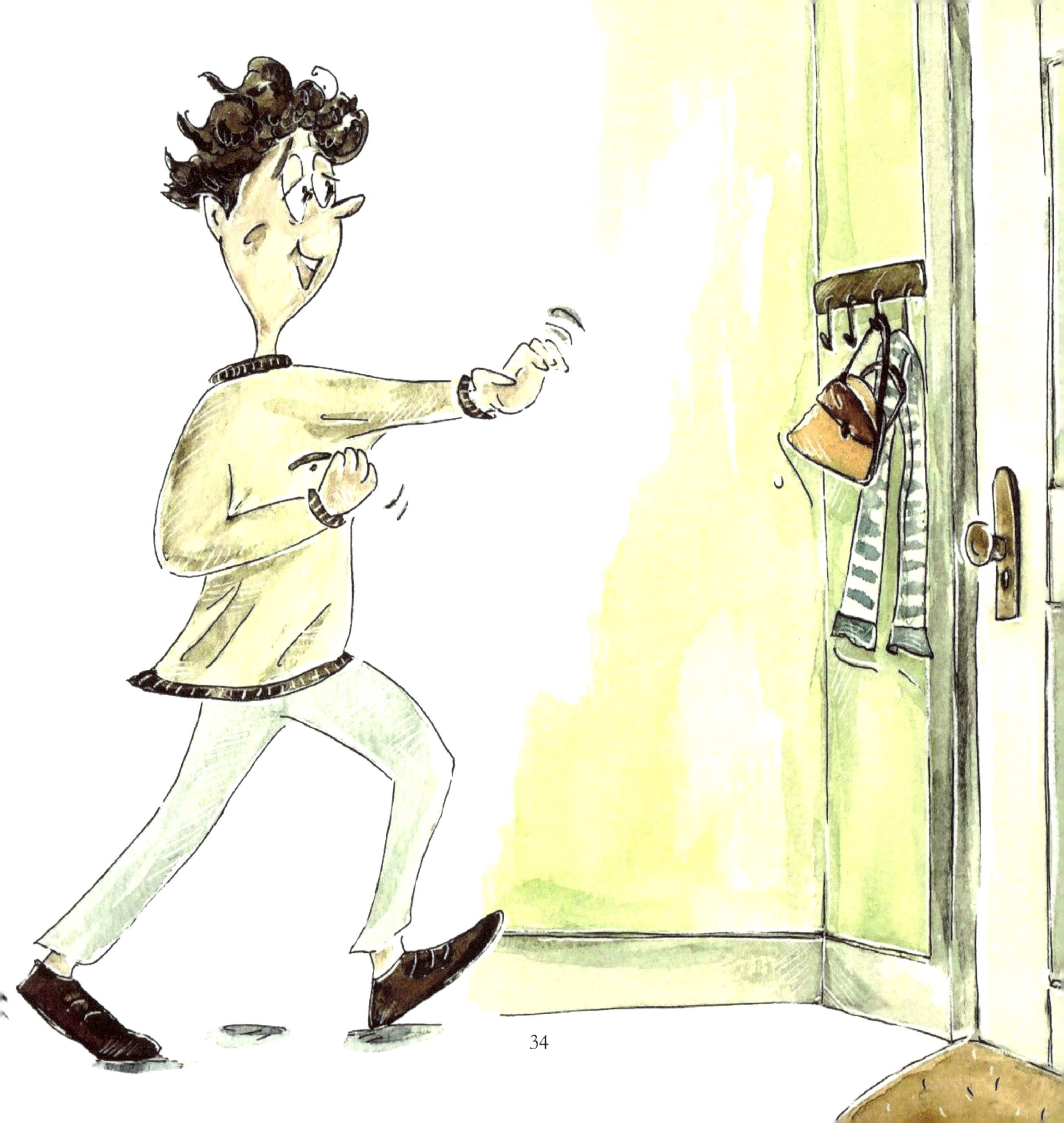

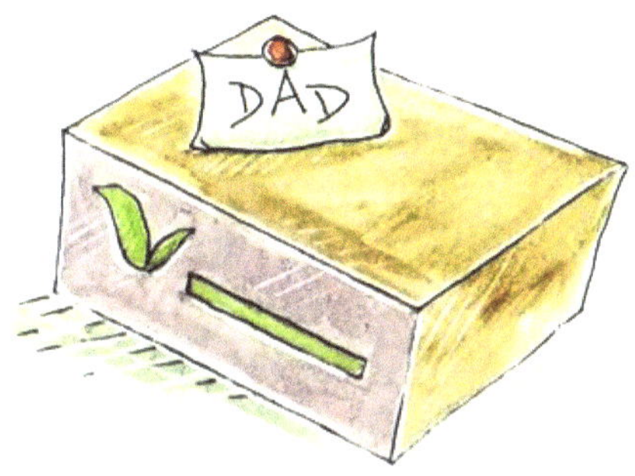

"I'm sorry I first thought your oils were silly," said Dad, sheepishly.

Knock, knock, knock!

"Excuse me you two, this one is for me!"

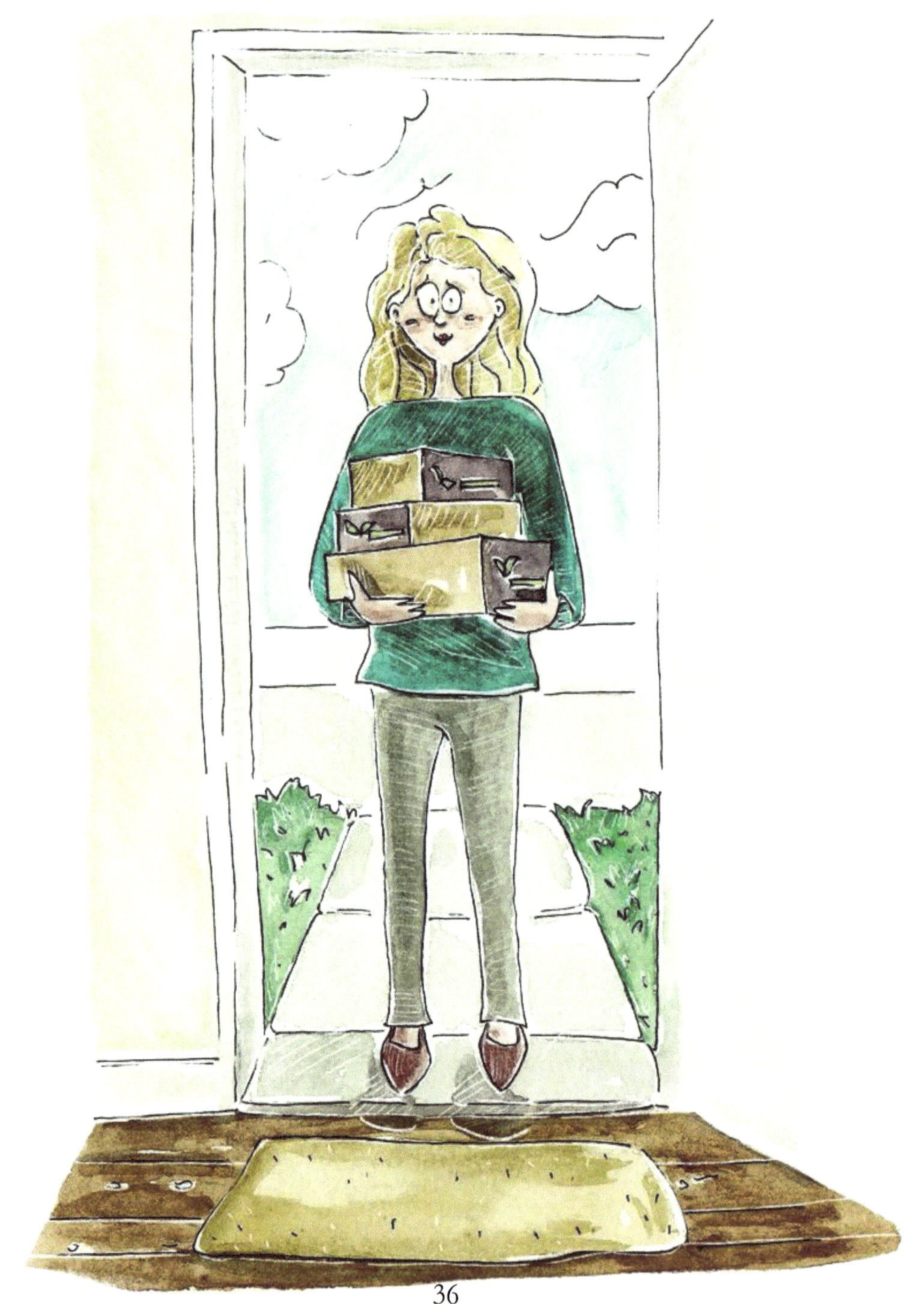

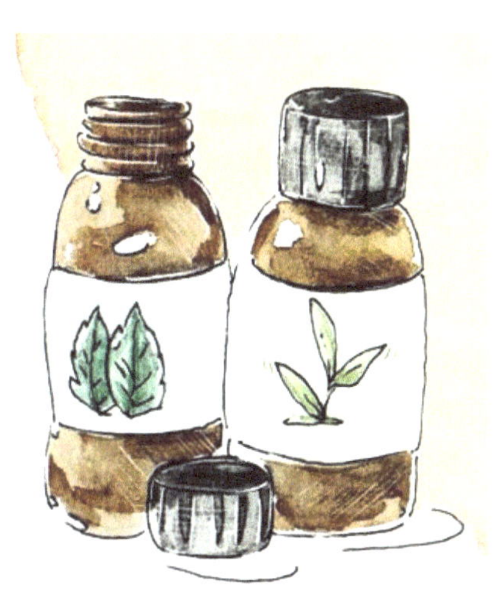

THE END

9 798581 812174